The Healing Power of Neem – Margosa

Time-tested Remedies for Common Ailments

Dueep Jyot Singh

Healthy Living Series

Mendon Cottage Books

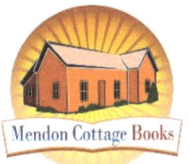

JD-Biz Publishing

Our books are available at

1. Amazon.com
2. Barnes and Noble
3. Itunes
4. Kobo
5. Smashwords
6. Google Play Books

Table of Contents

Introduction

The Neem- Azadirachta Indica – Margosa was an indigenous plant found in the Indian subcontinent, but thanks to more and more people all over the world knowing all about its miraculous long-term curative properties, it is being used as an alternative medicine cure by naturopaths globally.

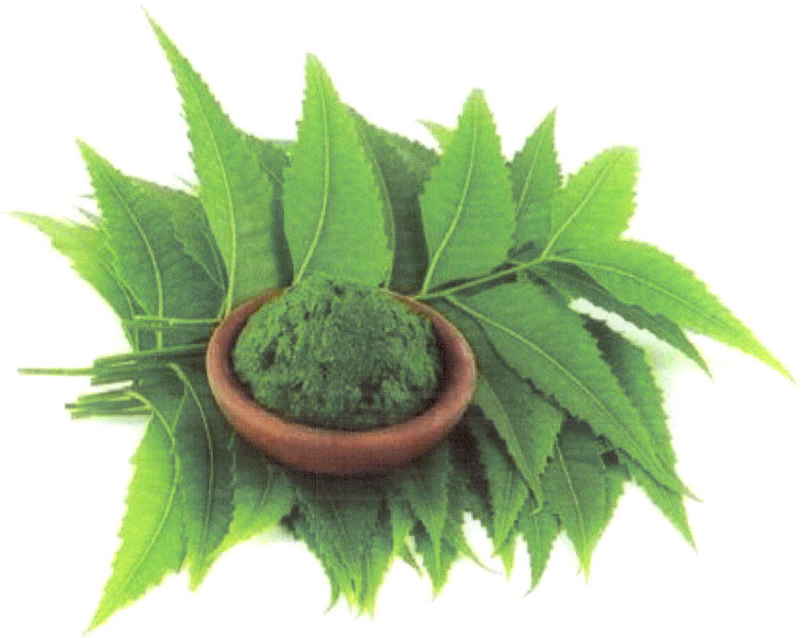

This book is going to tell you all about some known and some lesser-known remedies which you can use as an organic fertilizer, as a pesticide, and also to cure yourself.

It has been estimated that if we collect all the seeds produced by all the neem trees in the world annually, we are going to get 4,018,000 tons of valuable seed. The market value of the seeds themselves is about $50 million. Apart from that, the wood can bring in another $20 million.

Nevertheless, we would prefer our neem trees flourishing in our gardens, and providing us with shade, seeds and leaves to keep us and our family healthy. It is also going to provide a natural air purifier for us and ours.

Herbal skin Soap from the neem seeds is normally made with neem seed oil extract. The leftover husk remaining after the oil has been extracted is used as an organic fertilizer, as well as fodder for farm animals.

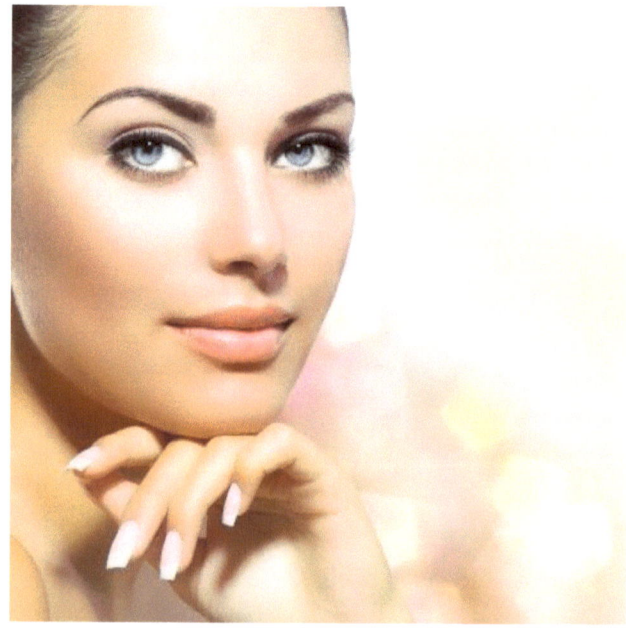

Lovely and flawless skin… She has been using herbal neem extract soap

A neem normally flowers in the summer. When we were young, my grandmother used to make sure that we never suffered from any sort of rainy season ailments including boils, diarrhea, or any other water borne diseases by giving us a decoction of fresh leaves every week. She took a fistful of fresh neem leaves, and boiled them in three glasses full of water.

It was terrible to drink because it was extremely bitter. But once it was down, we were given a spoonful of clarified butter in order to prevent the bitter leaves damaging our internal system if possible. And then we were given another spoonful of honey to get rid of the bitter taste.

She was only following the practice followed by her ancestors to keep the children healthy. Even father, all grown up had to drink this decoction, one small glass twice a week, even though he made "thoroughly disgusted" faces and told his mother firmly that he was not a child.

He was overruled. Nevertheless, this decoction made sure that we never suffered from skin diseases, stomach ailments or any other sort of disease, even when we grew up. Our immunity system was so strong by then.

Also, according to her, the neem leaves purified our blood, and it sure that we never suffered from any sort of blood related or mineral deficiency diseases including anemia, or even any blood cell infection diseases.

Neem seeds

A flowering neem tree, just before it fruits is going to feel the surrounding atmosphere with a very pleasant fragrance. The fruit is somewhat like a grape, green in color with a seed in it, surrounded by the pulp.

Some of the parts of a neem are bitter and somewhat sour in taste. These include the leaves. Each part of a neem tree is going to be used somewhere or the other, either as a medicine, or as wood. That means you are going to be using their flowers, leaves, bark and the fruit often, when you know to which use, you can put them.

This tree can grow to a height of 20 feet and more, when it is given lots of place in which to spread itself. My grandfather planted a neem tree outside the boundary wall of the house that he built in 1963. By 2003, the neem tree's branches had managed to creep under the boundary wall, and had begun to encroach into the garden, destroying the boundary wall in the process. That is why, the neem tree is never planted in an area surrounded by obstructions which it is going to grow under, within the next 50 years.

Curry trees

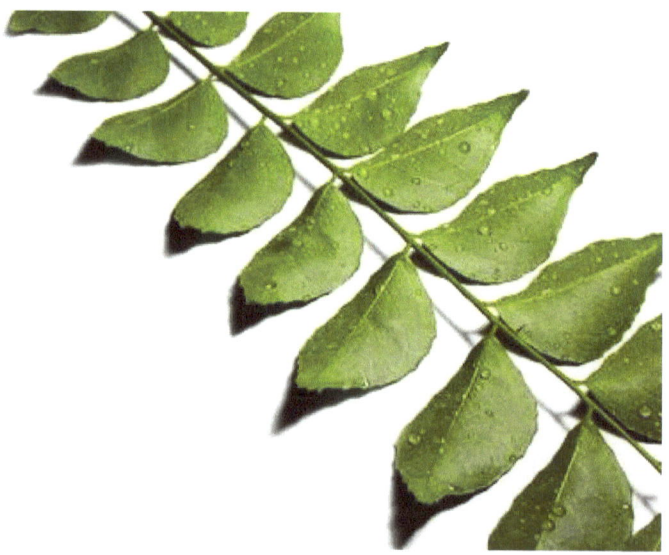

If you are living in the East and you do not have a curry plant in your garden, your garden is supposedly incomplete. That is the reason why I was rather amused when I saw a neighbor asking her gardener to plant a curry tree in the front of our house. She had obtained it from her brother's house, and not knowing much about gardening, she had plucked it from the ground, without bothering about the roots.

The poor silent gardener did not dare tell "Madam" that the tree would not grow. I being tactless did, and she told me that it was the rainy season and the tree would grow because she said so. I never argue with stubborn fools.

Apart from being used as a culinary delight, these curry leaves are excellent to cure diarrhea and dysentery. Take a fistful of these leaves, and make an infusion of it. Just half a cup of this infusion taken once a day is going to help cure this stomach infection. It is also going to get rid of cramps and pain in the stomach. The ordinary leaves are also effective enough to cure the stomach ailments, but who really wants to bother about bitter leaves drunk down?

Neem Paste for Skin Diseases

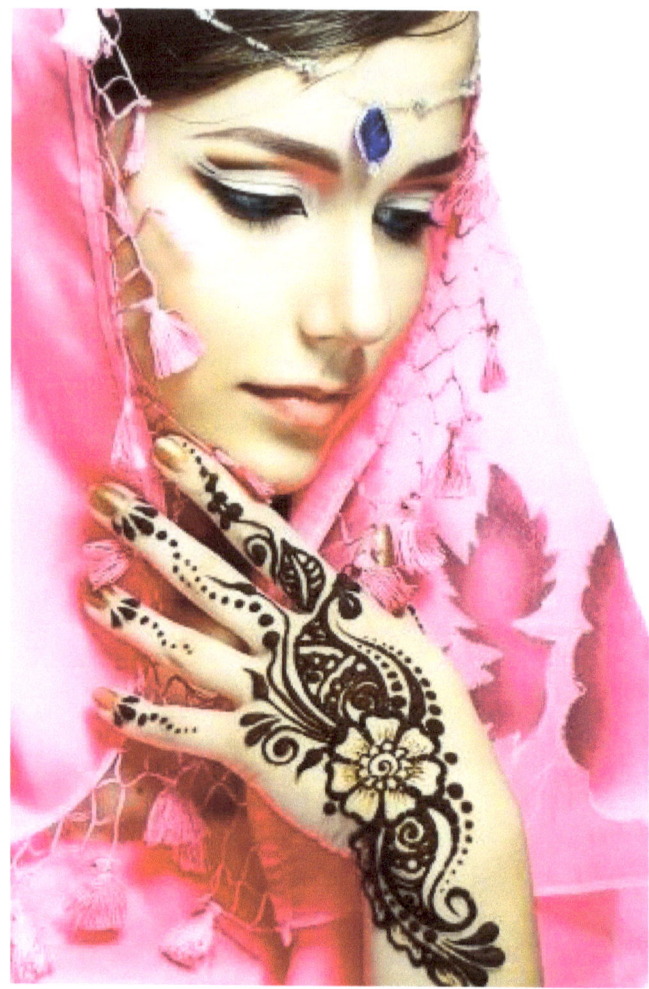

No pimples, no wrinkles…

Apart from the decoction, grandma also made a neem paste with around 679 grams of neem, mixed with 10 pepper Corns. This was ground together and spread all over the affected area, especially when one was suffer from skin diseases. This got rid of eczema, itching, boils, rashes and any sort of pimples or any affliction on the body's surface.

If you are suffering from pimples or even rashes or itch, here is one cure which I am going to suggest. Make a decoction of neem leaves and added to your bath water. You may want to include the neem leaves, also in the water, – you can always towel them off after your bath – and steep yourself in the neem leaf water.

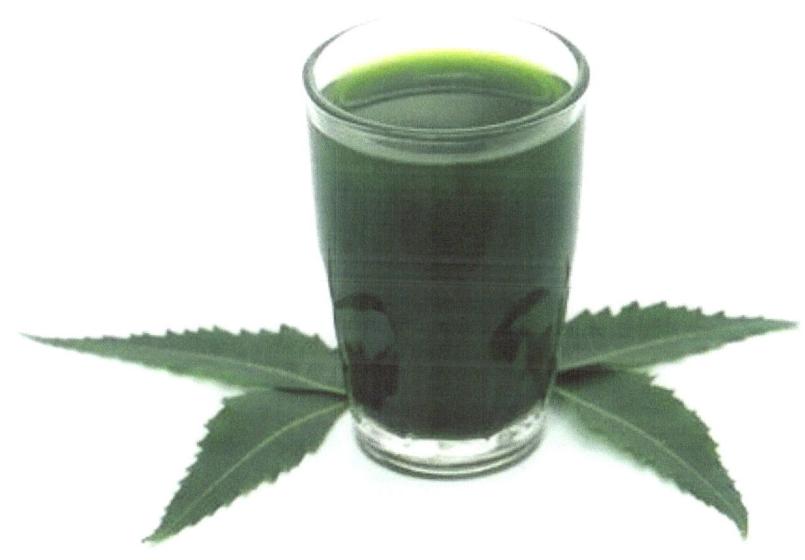

Wash away all the impurities naturally, and get out of your bath, feeling refreshed. Apart from this, your skin is going to feel rejuvenated and within the week, you are going to find yourself with a perfectly healthy skin.

In fact, this was used in ancient times to clean out infected wounds obtained during battle. The warriors just used to wash the blood away, and then apply a paste of neem leaves on the wound. 99.9% of the time, they were healed. The point. 1% was only if there was some foreign object left in the wound, which had not been removed during the initial washing which incidentally was done with neem water and honey.

Neem Flowers

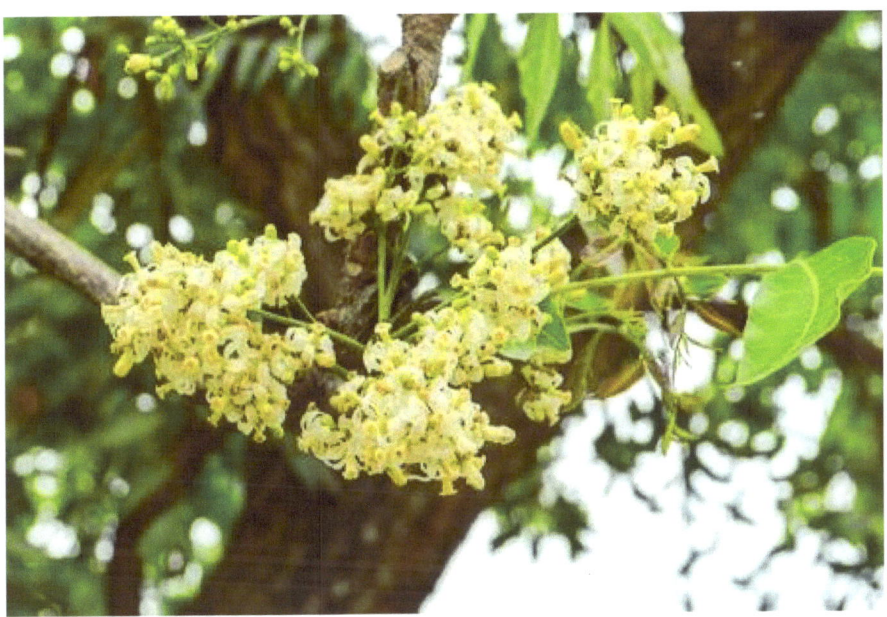

The flowers of the neem have also been used since ancient times to purify the blood. They are also used as an addition to curries and soups, in order to provide the resulting delicious dish with a subtle flavor.

There are two types of neem trees present in the Indian subcontinent. One has better leaves than one has sweet leaves. The one with sweet leaves is known as curry tree, even though it is the younger brother of the original bitter neem tree. Curry leaves are definitely a necessary part of Easton cuisine, where they are put either in fresh form or in dried form in curries, gravies, and in other liquid preparations.

Preparing a Soothing Eyeliner

Tell me about one beauty conscious lady in the world who does not like to line her eyes with some mysterious kohl, also known as kajal. Since time memorial, women in the East have been adding to the mystique of their eyes, by darkening and lining them.

Nowadays, you get these items in the market, inexpensive packages, with lots of amicable additives which are very harmful for your eyes. But centuries ago, ladies made kohl right at home, to keep the eyes of the family members healthy. This was made with neem bark, neem flowers or with neem leaves.

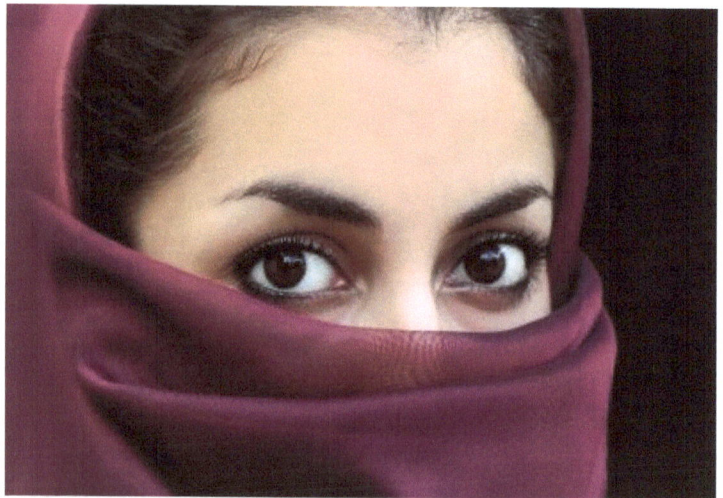

Here is one remedy I am going to tell you, when you suffer from irritation in the eyes, apart from beautifying them. Wrap up some neem flowers in a dab of cotton, and make it into a wick. Now place this wick in a lamp full of mustard oil. Now place a metal plate inverted over this lamp, and allow it to burn throughout the night.

I normally do this by placing the lamp between two bricks and then placing the metal plate upside down, covering the bricks. Do not allow the lamp light to touch the metal. It is going to discolor it. I ruined a copper plate, through this particular negligence. Now I have a copper plate with black and light blue defacing marks on its surface, due to the heat.

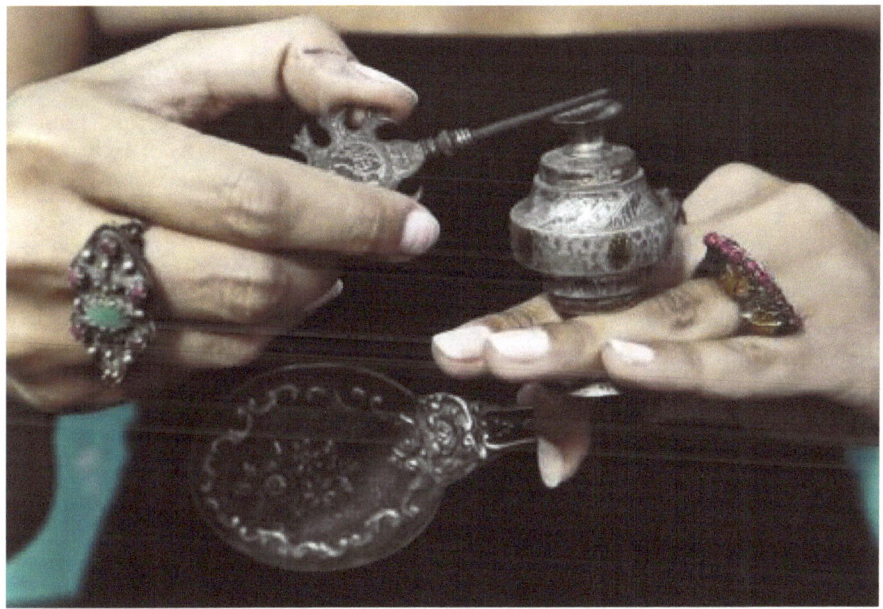

These Kohl bottles were normally made of silver in ancient times with silver applicators. I had one belonging to my grand mother and went online to look for its price. Well, it was just a cool $560! No thank you. Many families in the East End and in the Middle East have these bottles coming down as inherited heirlooms.

The next morning you are going to see a sooty deposit, all over the surface. This is the kohl, which you buy from the market. Just put this in a small glass jar, and mix it with either some rosewater, or with some clarified butter to make it into a spreadable paste. Apply it to your eyes with a Q-tip.

Now remember that this is not only antiseptic, but it is also going to be so dark that it is going to remain beautifying your eyes for a large number of hours. That is why I apply it at night before going to sleep. By the morning, the excess of kohl is washed away, and I have a beautiful outline which is going to last me throughout the day.

You may say that your eyes water a bit, when you apply the kohl. That is because the clarified butter is clearing out your tear ducts. It is going to happen for the first two or three applications, but then your eyes are going to get to this new natural healthy beauty product.

Irritation in Your Eyes

If you want to get rid of the irritation in your eyes, you are not going to add clarified butter. Instead, you are going to add 0.70 g of roasted powdered alum, and 20 g of unsalted butter. [If you make it at home, so much the better, because then you are not going to worry about preservatives. That is why clarified butter was used in ancient times.] Mix the kohl in it to make a paste. The alum is to get rid of any sort of infection in your eyes. The butter is to prevent your eyes from smarting.

The ladies in ancient times did not have a Q-tip with which to apply this kohl in their eyes, so they just used a dainty stem off the neem tree itself. This is also a good remedy for the regrowth of the eyelashes, if they are sparse and have fallen off.

Eye Wash

There is also another traditional remedy, which is known as the neem eyewash. Take a few handfuls of neem leaves and dry them in the sun. When they are completely dry, just powder them and place them in a clay utensil.

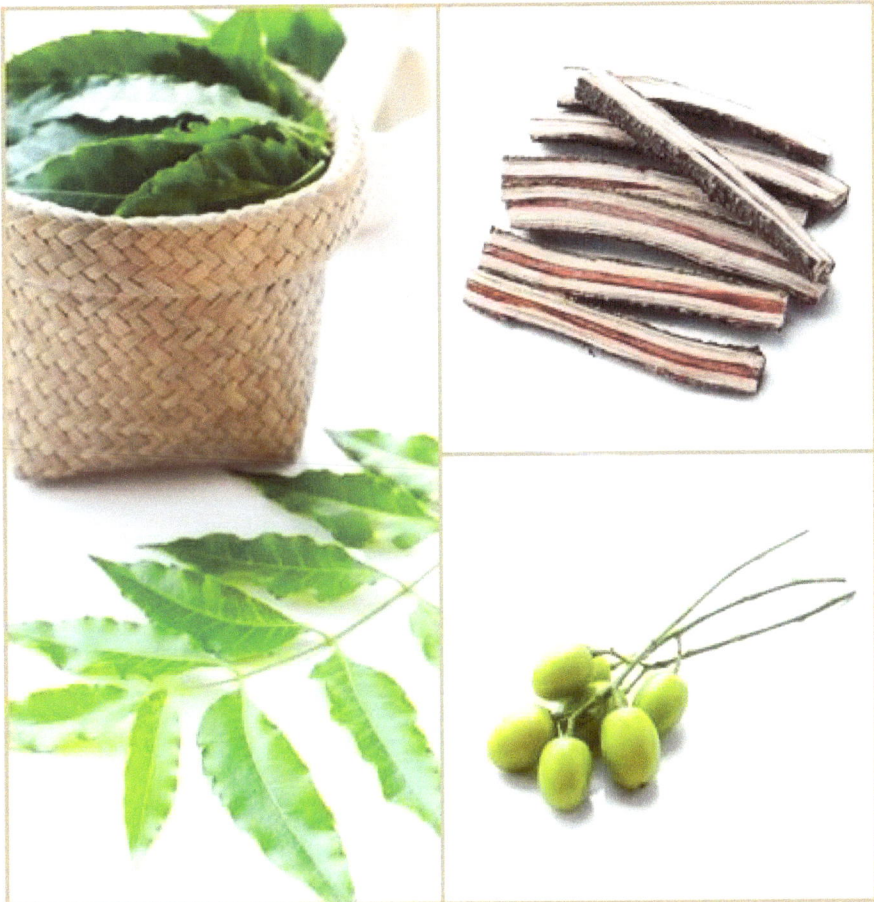

As this is an ancient remedy, and at that time, metal utensils were not so very common with the common people, clay utensils were used for cooking. Anyway, put it on the heat, along with the neem leaves, until they are charred. Take out the powder and add some lemon juice water in the mixture. Make a semiliquid paste and put it in a glass bottle.

This is the best eyewash which you would ever get to get rid of any irritation in the eyes, infection or any sort of problems in your eyes. Just dip an applicator in this mixture, and apply it into your eyes morning and evening. It is going to smart a little, because of the lemon juice water, but this is the reason why so many ancients had clear vision even when they were in their 90th decade and more.

In the same way, you can also put one drop of fresh neem juice in your eyes. If they are aching or irritating you, the initial smarting is going to cool down the ache. But if you want to cure your child of eye irritation, do not put this juice in their eyes. Instead put two drops in their ears. Surprisingly enough, if there is only one eye aching, you put two drops in the opposite ear.

Neem Remedies

Apart from this plant being used for skin diseases as well as a blood purifier, neem has been used down the centuries for a number of other purposes.

For Stroke Victims

I have seen this in action. The right side of an acquaintance was paralyzed due to a stroke and his wife obtained some fresh neem oil from the neem seeds in the garden. [That was extracted from the town's mill.] The affected region was massaged vigorously, 3 to 4 times a day without fail. Within three weeks, there was a visible improvement in that area, and the muscles had begun to respond to stimuli.

I do not know why research has not been done on this particular field, especially for stroke patients. It is a pity, especially when their condition could be improved beneficially with regular massages.

In Kipling's Rewards and Fairies, Simple Simon, a friend of Sir Francis Drake was injured fighting the Spaniards and was restored due to massage.

'The Spanisher gave us his broadside as he went about. They all fell short except one that smack-smooth hit the rail behind my back, an' I felt most won'erful cold.

'"Be you hit anywhere to signify?" he says. "Come over to me."

'"O Lord, Mus' Drake," I says, "my legs won't move," and that was the last I spoke for months.'

'Why? What had happened?' cried Dan and Una together.

'The rail had jarred me in here like.' Simon reached behind him clumsily. 'From my shoulders down I didn't act no shape. Frankie carried me piggyback to my Aunt's house, and I lay bed-rid and tongue-tied while she rubbed me day and night, month in and month out. She had faith in rubbing with the hands. P'raps she put some of her gifts into it, too. Last of all, something loosed itself in my pore back, and lo! I was whole restored again, but kitten-feeble.

If wise women knew about the power of massage in the days of the Spanish Armada, it is still relevant in the 21st century.

Flatulence and Dyspepsia

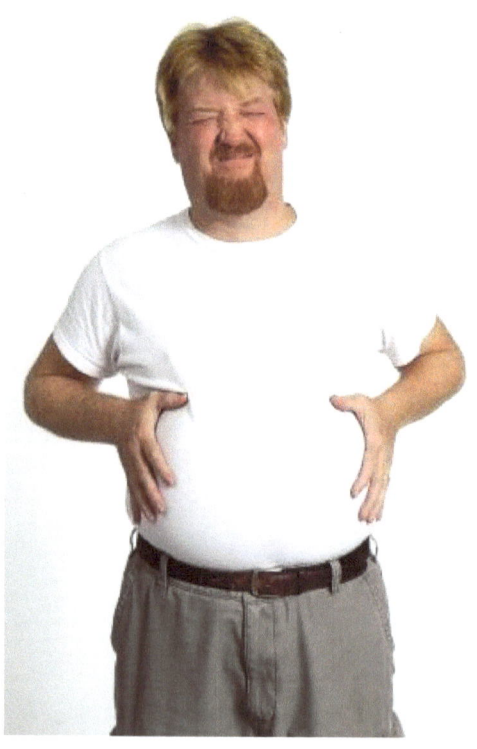

Flatulence and dyspepsia are some of the side effects of an unregulated diet. So if you are suffering from any sort of these particular stomach ailments, all you have to do is chew up on some of the ripe neem fruit. Do not eat the seeds but swallow the pulp. This is going to clear up your system wonderfully well and make you feel hungry again.

Constipation

If you are suffering from constipation, all you have to do is take 10 g of fresh neem leaves, and grind them. Add them to a glassful of water. Drink this up first thing in the morning and you are going to find your system cleared within half an hour. If you want, you can also add a little bit of rock candy as well as three – four peppercorns for taste.

Piles

It seems that the pulp from fresh right neem fruit is excellent for curing piles. Just take 2 tablespoons full of this pulp and mix it in one glass of water. Drink this 3 to 4 times a day, until you are cured completely.

Fumigation

I remember spending a summer, in a town, where the summer had brought in lots of mosquitoes and flies. The people in that town were so used to the mosquitoes and flies, that they did not bother much about them, saying that these were usual, especially in the heat. That was when I got really annoyed, because closing the windows meant a really hot room, without any air conditioning.

So I just gathered some twigs with dried neem leaves, which were under any tree. Lucky for me, they were there, otherwise I would have to wait for another week in order to get those twigs to dry.

I just made them into a torch and lit them in my room, after shutting the doors and windows. This fumigation with the powerful odor of neem had everyone in the vicinity pouring in, – even with the shut doors and windows – to find out what I was up to and how potentially dangerous it was to the spectators. The fumes got rid of all the mosquitoes and the flies, to their great amazement.

Also, the room had begun to smell really nice and fresh. So now whenever I go to that town, I am so glad to see it completely mosquito and fly free. I am surprised that more people do not use this natural fumigation method to get rid of pests. Instead, they buy poisonous pesticides and room fresheners, which give their children respiratory problems.

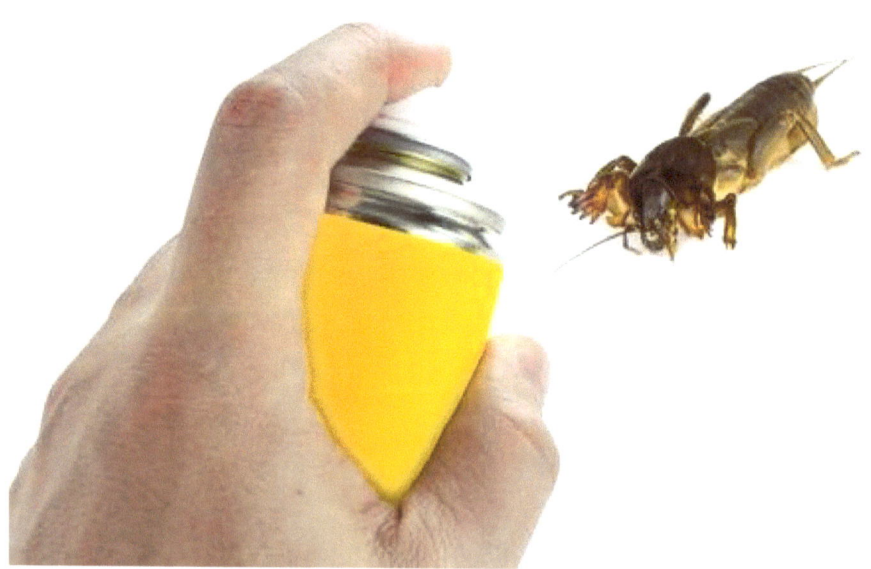

This can be done without resorting to chemical fumigants.

In the same way, my room was infested with a large number of bedbugs, which my hosts considered to be normal, because according to them, where there was furniture there would be bedbugs. Talk about being foolish martyrs to convention. I just requested them to get a little bit of yellow powdered sulfur from the market, and collected some neem leaves from the garden. And then I lit the funeral pyre of the bedbugs.

Talk about hundred percent fumigation. 20 g of sulfur, five handfuls of neem leaves and a matchstick. Then we went outside and shut the door behind us. The sulfur was enough to stink up the atmosphere for the next eight hours, and we had to open the windows to get rid of the fumes. But all the bedbugs were dead, never to reappear again.

I hear that there is a sulfur based chemical gas called Vikane used for the treatment of bedbugs by pesticide companies. Do not use chemicals.

Malaria and Periodic Fever Cure

Here is another lesser known facts about neem, which people do not know. Before cinchona was found out to be an effective remedy for malaria and periodic fever, people in the East had been using it a decoction of neem bark in water given to the patient three times everyday to get rid of the infection.

Dr. Ross, who finally recognized the role of the malarial germ carrying female Anopheles mosquito, in the swamps of India did not notice the fact that British soldiers and officers often fell prey to malaria, every year, and suffered greatly. Until of course he taught them to eat cinchona tablets to prevent malaria. On the other hand, the native soldiers never suffered from malaria, because their wives and mothers fed them neem bark, taken from inside of the neem tree decoctions every evening. To this mixture, they added a bit of dried ginger powder and red chili powder to counteract the very powerful effect of the bark.

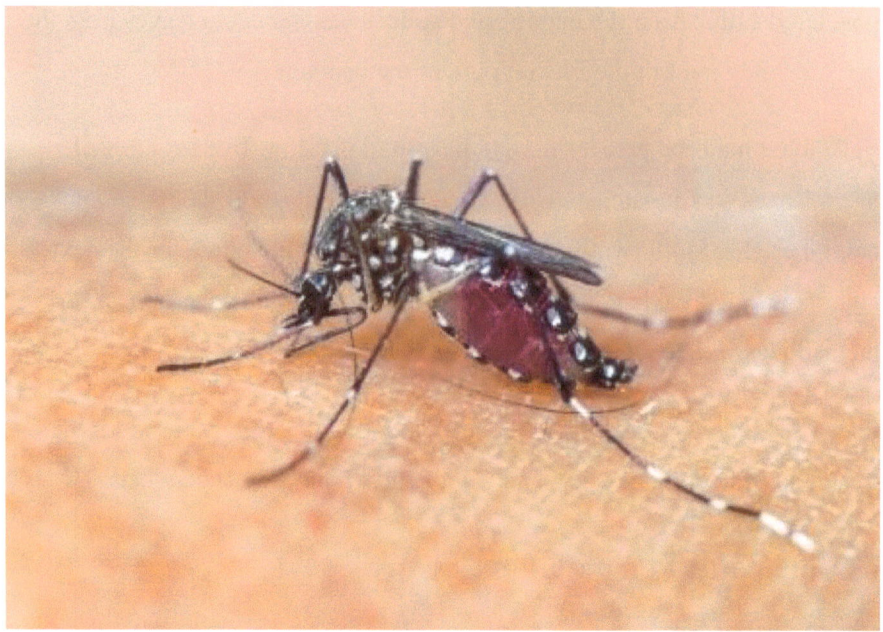

So anybody who wants to do some research on how malaria and periodic fevers are prevented through neem bark can waste plenty of the taxpayers money on something which is well known since ancient times.

However, if they come to the remote villages of the Indian subcontinent where there are no doctors around, and they happen to fall sick, they are immediately going to be put in a room fumigated with neem leaves, and are going to be fed a ground mixture of fresh neem leaves and stems in water, until the fever leaves them.

My Natural Oil Remedy

Now this is a remedy, which can be made by any wise woman and placed in her medicine cupboard. Take about 50 fresh leaves of the neem, and soak it in 250 g of your favorite oil. Allow to boil, until the leaves are burned completely. Filter into a glass bottle, and use whenever you suffer from cuts, wounds, and even burns.

Oil Ointment

Here is the oil ointment which I make every winter with 250 g neem oil, 125 g wax, and one Kg juice of fresh neem leaves. To this I add 50 g of powder neem bark and 25 g of neem leaves ashes.

Put the juice and oil on low heat until the amount is reduced to half. To this, you are now going to add the wax. After you have mixed it well, add the powdered bark and the ash of the leaves to the mixture. Place this ointment in a glass jar. It is going to keep for a really long while and make sure that you never suffer from any infected wounds, cuts, scrapes, burns, or any other sort of painful injuries.

Sprains

I nearly forgot about this particular remedy, which was used on me, once when I was a child, by surprisingly enough, my physical training teacher! I fell down while playing dodgeball, – the opposite team hated me because they never knew which way I would jump – and I landed badly, spraining my leg and ankle.

A sprain especially in the ankle or in the knee is very painful, and my teacher immediately applied a lotion, which he had prepared and had kept in his locker. It was made up of mustard oil in which a few fresh neem leaves had been boiled and burned. To this was added a little bit of turmeric powder.

This lotion/oil was immediately spread all over my sprain, with the rest of my classmates watching the proceedings very eagerly. This was then bandaged tight. Believe it or not, within three hours, I was ready to walk home.

Naturally, all of us came home, and asked our parents and grandparents to make this oil immediately and keep it ready for sprains. This oil keeps up to six months, because the turmeric starts to decompose during this time.

Prickly Heat

I remember going on a holiday, and forgetting to pack my bottle of prickly heat powder. When I got down from the plane, the muggy atmosphere of my new destination was enough to have me suffering badly from this irritating condition.

Luckily, my hosts had a neem tree growing in their garden. I immediately had a bath with neem leaves added to the water. After that, I applied neem oil all over the affected area. This condition vanished within 30 – 48 hours. So now I always forget about my prickly heat powder as long as I have neem oil with me.

Joint Pain

Any sort of joint pain can be gotten rid of by just grinding the inner bark of the neem, with a little bit of water. Apply this paste on the affected regions. You are going to find relief within a couple of days after you have been applying this paste three – four times a day to the affected areas.

Different Uses of Neem

Apart from neem being a medical boon to help take care of your health throughout your life, it has also been used for centuries for a number of other uses, including pesticides and fodder.

My grandmother used to place neem leaves under warm clothes, in books, in cupboards and in any other place, where she was afraid of termites, mold, fungus, mites, moths and silverfish. She had learned to do this from her elders in a time when there were no mothballs and naphthalene balls in existence.

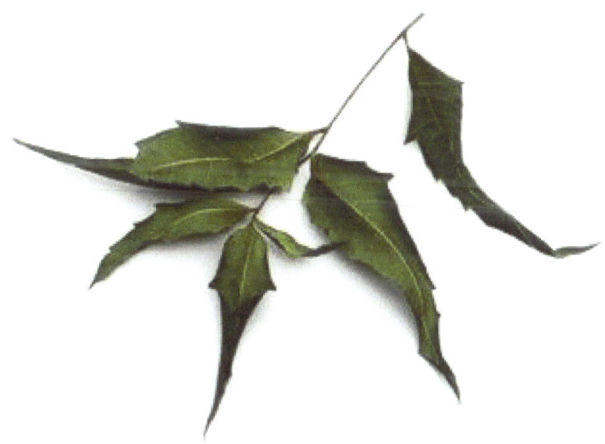

These are sun-dried neem leaves. They are excellent for preserving your valuable items from moths, mildew, fungus, and silverfish.

Grandma would pluck a large number of neem leaves, and dry them in the sun, in shade. This would take about a week. The sun – drying, especially in the shade was essential, because direct sunlight would get rid of all the important essential and powerful neem oil, thus rendering the leaves useless.

The neem leaves were then collected, and then placed on a cloth, in a layer. After that, the clothes to be preserved, especially woollens, silks , brocades and other expensive garments were placed on top of the neem leaves, and the outer cloth wrapping the clothes.

She normally turned out the clothes every two – three years, to put in another new handful of dried neem leaves. She had clothes more than half a century old, and still fresh and new looking. And that was because there was absolutely no chance of any moths getting to the woolens and silks.

In the same way, any termite infested area in the gardens was immediately treated to an organic fertilizer of neem leaves and crushed neem seeds. This would immediately get rid of all the pests, including the termites and the ants.

Pesticides

Here is an ancient natural pesticide, which is going to get rid of all the pests, as well as make sure that your food is not poisoned with poisonous chemicals. Take 50 L of water and dissolve one liter of neem oil in it. Use this pesticide spraying all over your plants, trees and other greenery. This natural organic pesticide is excellent to protect your plants from pests.

Do the spraying after you have planted them, and once mid-way, while they are growing and just before fruiting.

Fodder for Poultry

Believe it or not, the seeds of the neem are one of the most proteinaceous food fodder that you could give to your poultry. You are going to also see an increase in their egg laying capacities. I saw an experimental farm using ground peanut husk from which the peanut oil had been extracted and neem seed husk. Along with that, they added lots of dried fish meal and greens to the fodder.

The eggs were larger in size, and really tasty.

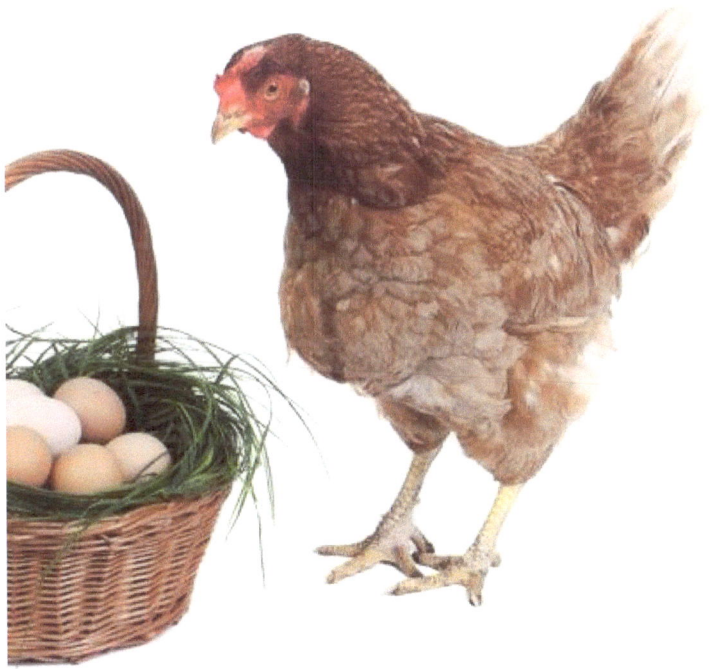

Neem Oil

If you want to purify your blood, or you want to get rid of all the parasites in your stomach, all you have to do is pop in some ripe neem fruit in your mouth and chew the pulp. It has a sweetish taste. The pulp is also considered to be an excellent cure for skin diseases. In fact, in ancient times, people took 70 g of neem pulp every day, drinking it down to get rid of possible leprosy and skin diseases. They continued this until they were cured completely.

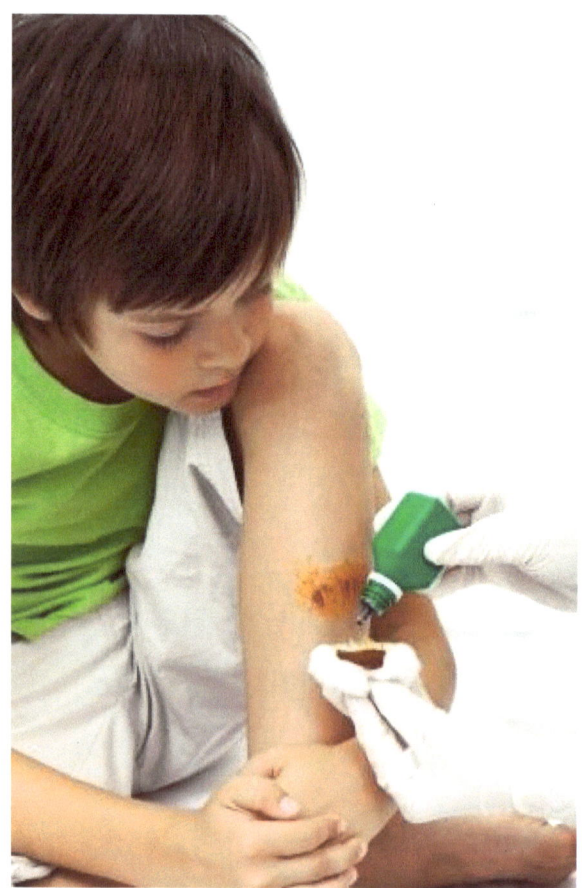

The seeds, when spat out on any ground are going to give rise to new neem trees. However, they are collected, and neem oil is extracted from them.

Neem oil is one of the products which is placed in an easily accessible place in my medical cabinet. I cannot do without it, because I use this as an antiseptic instead of Dettol or Savlon. And the good thing is, even though I may be hurt rather badly, application of the oil means that I am not going to scar.

When I was suffering from otitis externa as a child, with fungal infections causing plenty of pain and infection in my ear, my grandmother kept looking for neem trees in the vicinity. According to her, all she had to do was to get out some neem oil, add some honey to it, and then dip a cotton earbud in it to clean my ear. That would have got rid of all the infection. That is what she did to her children and grandchildren.

But as there were no neem trees present, she got rid of that infection by heating up some mustard oil and putting two cloves of crushed garlic in it. After that she put two warm eardrops in my infected ears, thrice a day and thus got rid of all that infection forever and ever.

Here is one remedy I found just by chance. I had just put on a pair of formal shoes, and had gone to an office of meeting. Unfortunately, those shoes had not been broken in, and by the time the meeting was over, my poor feet were weeping with pain. Also, there had been blisters forming on my toes as well as at the back of my ankles, which had been sorely chafed by the Socks, whenever I walked and moved my feet.

So I took them off gingerly when I came back home, added some neem oil to some melted wax and applied this mixture all over my blisters and draw chafed spots. After that I did not have to worry about the skin rubbing away because the socks protected the skin with its wax covering.

I also applied some ordinary coconut oil to the leather, where it was chafing, and rubbed it in to make the leather more supple. After that, I put the shoes out in the sun for about an hour so that the oil could get absorbed in the leather. Two days of this treatment and the shoe was broken in. I have been wearing those shoes for the last six years without any problems and they have traveled miles and miles, without making my feet feel tormented and tortured.

Conclusion

Thanks to the known benefits of the neem, I have been in the habit of eating five little leaves of the neem tree, ever since I was a child. That meant I never suffered from throat infections, mouth or gum problems, halitosis, and other problems.

When I had some official meetings scheduled for a particular day, and I knew that I did not want to embarrass myself with bad breath, I began washing my mouth out with neem water – neem leaves boiled in water – thrice a day and even gargling with it to get rid of any possible infection.

Within four days, there was absolutely no chance of bad breath, and that is why it did not have to worry about mouth fresheners and Listerine. So now this neem water infusion is made every week, placed in a bottle in the bathroom, and after I brush my teeth, I do the gargling and most freshening with a mouthful of this liquid. And I do not have to worry about halitosis ever.

So, you may want to know how the ancients treated wounds with neem? First of all, the leaves were boiled in about 750 g of water, to make a neem solution. This was then dribbled all over the wound to clean it out of any sort of blood, dirt and other impurities. After that, the wound was "dried" by the placing of a clean piece of cotton cloth over it.

The cotton cloth was removed, the moment it got damp. That meant that all the water content on the wound had been absorbed in the cloth and now it was ready for the placing of an ointment. The ointment was applied and the hurt bandaged again with another bandage. This healed the wound, which was inspected every morning for the replacement of the bandage on the injury after cleaning and putting on fresh ointment.

So now you say, you have nearly finished the book, but how, I did not tell you how you would plant a neem in your own garden? Neem has been cultivated in the USA especially in nurseries in southern Florida. And because it needs a subtropical or a tropical atmosphere, you can grow it without any problem in California, Texas and Arizona too. It needs a zone 10, in which to grow.

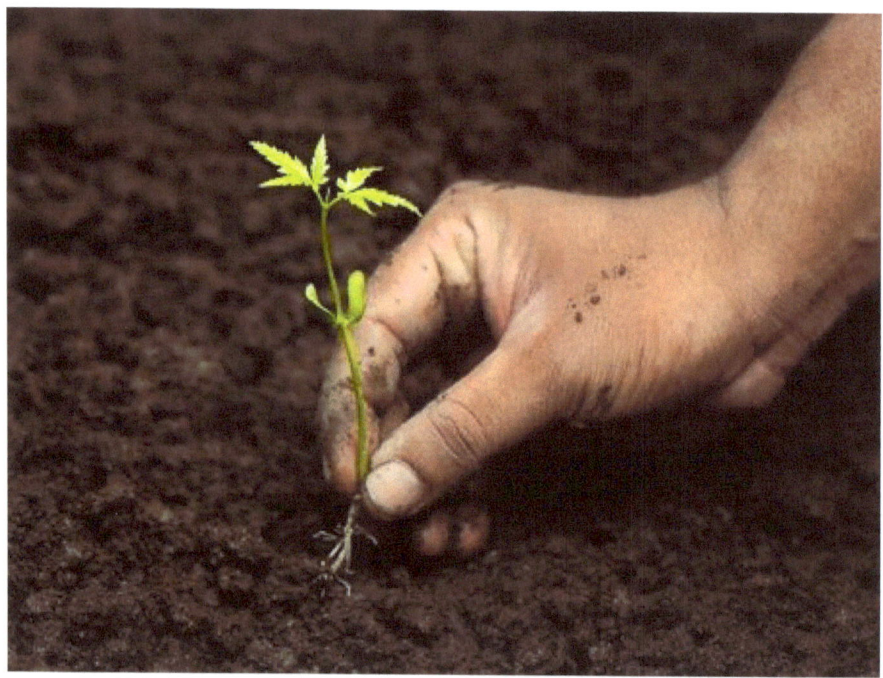

You may find this URL interesting reading.

http://www.ncnhdistrict.org/aom/neem.html

Neem is now being grown all over the world, and the potential for it to be grown commercially is slowly and steadily being acknowledged by many horticulturalists.

So take full advantage of this natural bounty, Live Long and Prosper!

Author Bio

Dueep Jyot Singh is a Management and IT Professional who managed to gather Postgraduate qualifications in Management and English and Degrees in Science, French and Education while pursuing different enjoyable career options like being an hospital administrator, IT,SEO and HRD Database Manager/ trainer, movie , radio and TV scriptwriter, theatre artiste and public speaker, lecturer in French, Marketing and Advertising, ex-Editor of Hearts On Fire (now known as Solstice) Books Missouri USA, advice columnist and cartoonist, publisher and Aviation School trainer, ex-moderator on Medico.in, banker, student councilor ,travelogue writer … among other things!

One fine morning, she decided that she had enough of killing herself by Degrees and went back to her first love -- writing. It's more enjoyable! She already has 48 published academic and 14 fiction- in- different- genre books under her belt.

When she is not designing websites or making Graphic design illustrations for clients , she is browsing through old bookshops hunting for treasures, of which she has an enviable collection – including R.L. Stevenson, O.Henry, Dornford Yates, Maurice Walsh, De Maupassant, Victor Hugo, Sapper, C.N. Williamson, "Bartimeus" and the crown of her collection- Dickens "The Old Curiosity Shop," and "Martin Chuzzlewit" and so on… Just call her "Renaissance Woman" - collecting herbal remedies, acting like Universal Helping Hand/Agony Aunt, or escaping to her dear mountains for a bit of exploring, collecting herbs and plants, and trekking.

Check out some of the other JD-Biz Publishing books

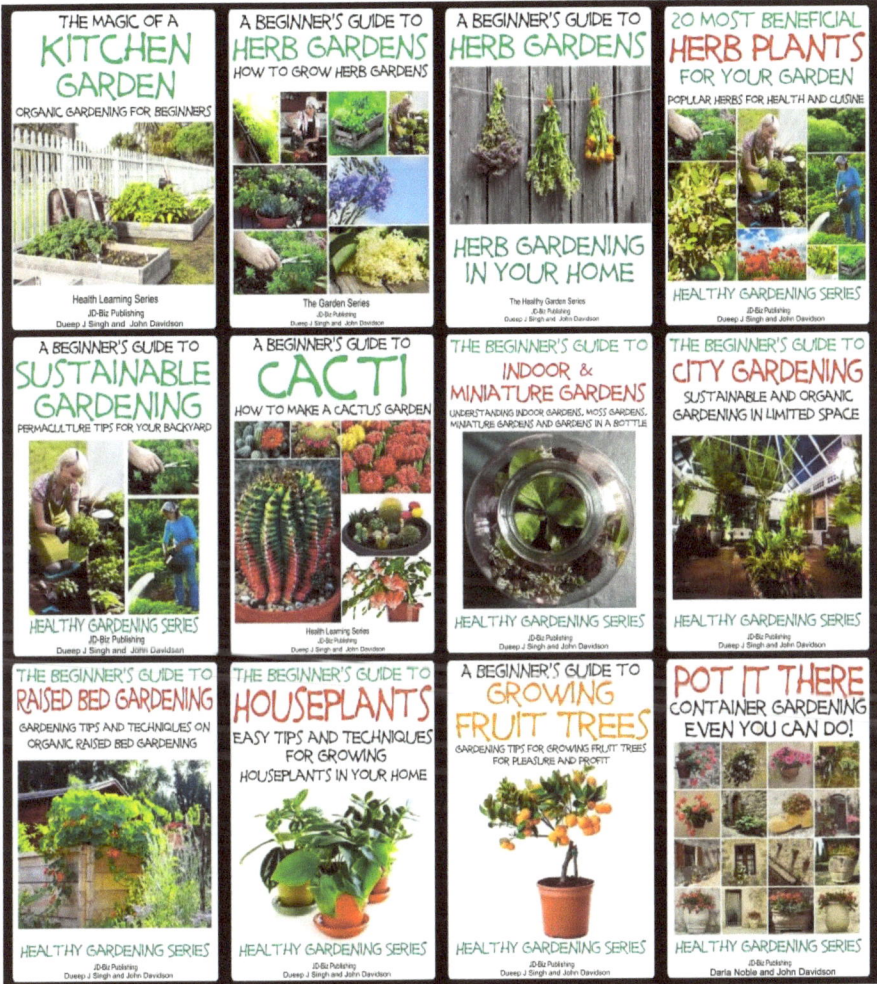

Health Learning Series

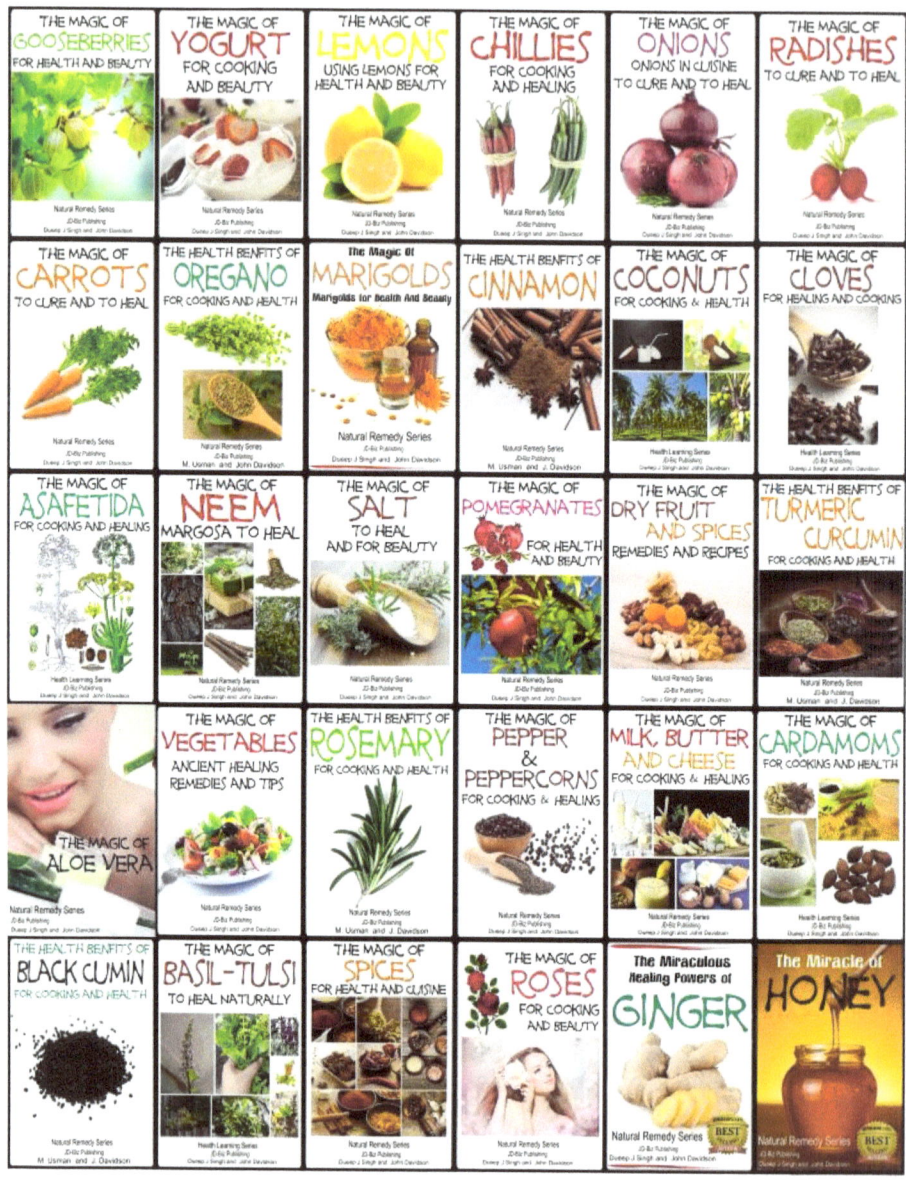

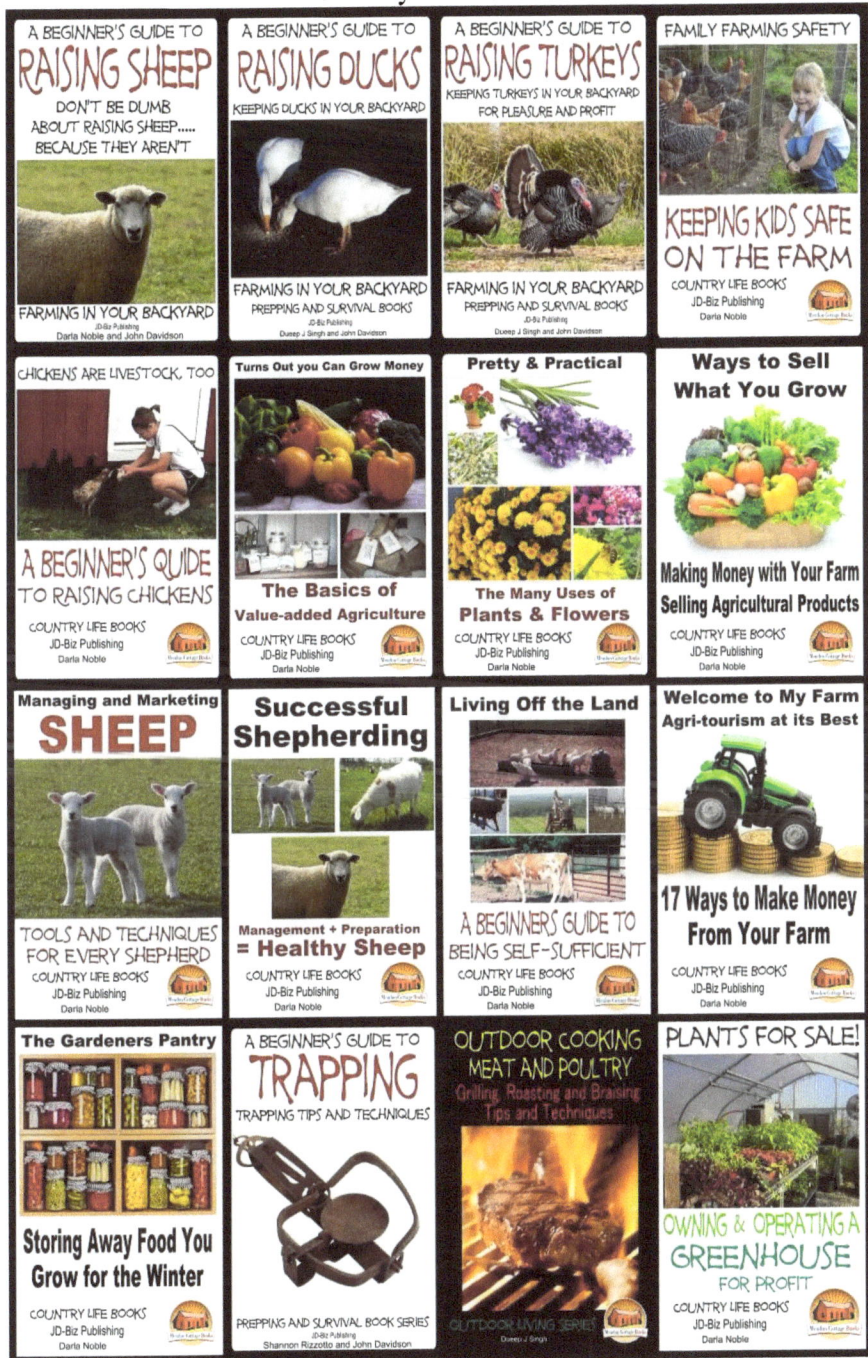

Row 1:
- A BEGINNER'S GUIDE TO RAISING SHEEP - DON'T BE DUMB ABOUT RAISING SHEEP..... BECAUSE THEY AREN'T - FARMING IN YOUR BACKYARD - JD-Biz Publishing - Darla Noble and John Davidson
- A BEGINNER'S GUIDE TO RAISING DUCKS - KEEPING DUCKS IN YOUR BACKYARD - FARMING IN YOUR BACKYARD - PREPPING AND SURVIVAL BOOKS - JD-Biz Publishing - Dueep J Singh and John Davidson
- A BEGINNER'S GUIDE TO RAISING TURKEYS - KEEPING TURKEYS IN YOUR BACKYARD FOR PLEASURE AND PROFIT - FARMING IN YOUR BACKYARD - PREPPING AND SURVIVAL BOOKS - JD-Biz Publishing - Dueep J Singh and John Davidson
- FAMILY FARMING SAFETY - KEEPING KIDS SAFE ON THE FARM - COUNTRY LIFE BOOKS - JD-Biz Publishing - Darla Noble

Row 2:
- CHICKENS ARE LIVESTOCK, TOO - A BEGINNER'S GUIDE TO RAISING CHICKENS - COUNTRY LIFE BOOKS - JD-Biz Publishing - Darla Noble
- Turns Out you Can Grow Money - The Basics of Value-added Agriculture - COUNTRY LIFE BOOKS - JD-Biz Publishing - Darla Noble
- Pretty & Practical - The Many Uses of Plants & Flowers - COUNTRY LIFE BOOKS - JD-Biz Publishing - Darla Noble
- Ways to Sell What You Grow - Making Money with Your Farm Selling Agricultural Products - COUNTRY LIFE BOOKS - JD-Biz Publishing - Darla Noble

Row 3:
- Managing and Marketing SHEEP - TOOLS AND TECHNIQUES FOR EVERY SHEPHERD - COUNTRY LIFE BOOKS - JD-Biz Publishing - Darla Noble
- Successful Shepherding - Management + Preparation = Healthy Sheep - COUNTRY LIFE BOOKS - JD-Biz Publishing
- Living Off the Land - A BEGINNER'S GUIDE TO BEING SELF-SUFFICIENT - COUNTRY LIFE BOOKS - JD-Biz Publishing - Darla Noble
- Welcome to My Farm Agri-tourism at its Best - 17 Ways to Make Money From Your Farm - COUNTRY LIFE BOOKS - JD-Biz Publishing - Darla Noble

Row 4:
- The Gardeners Pantry - Storing Away Food You Grow for the Winter - COUNTRY LIFE BOOKS - JD-Biz Publishing - Darla Noble
- A BEGINNER'S GUIDE TO TRAPPING - TRAPPING TIPS AND TECHNIQUES - PREPPING AND SURVIVAL BOOK SERIES - JD-Biz Publishing - Shannon Rizzotto and John Davidson
- OUTDOOR COOKING MEAT AND POULTRY - Grilling, Roasting and Braising Tips and Techniques - OUTDOOR LIVING SERIES - Dueep J Singh
- PLANTS FOR SALE! - OWNING & OPERATING A GREENHOUSE FOR PROFIT - COUNTRY LIFE BOOKS - JD-Biz Publishing - Darla Noble

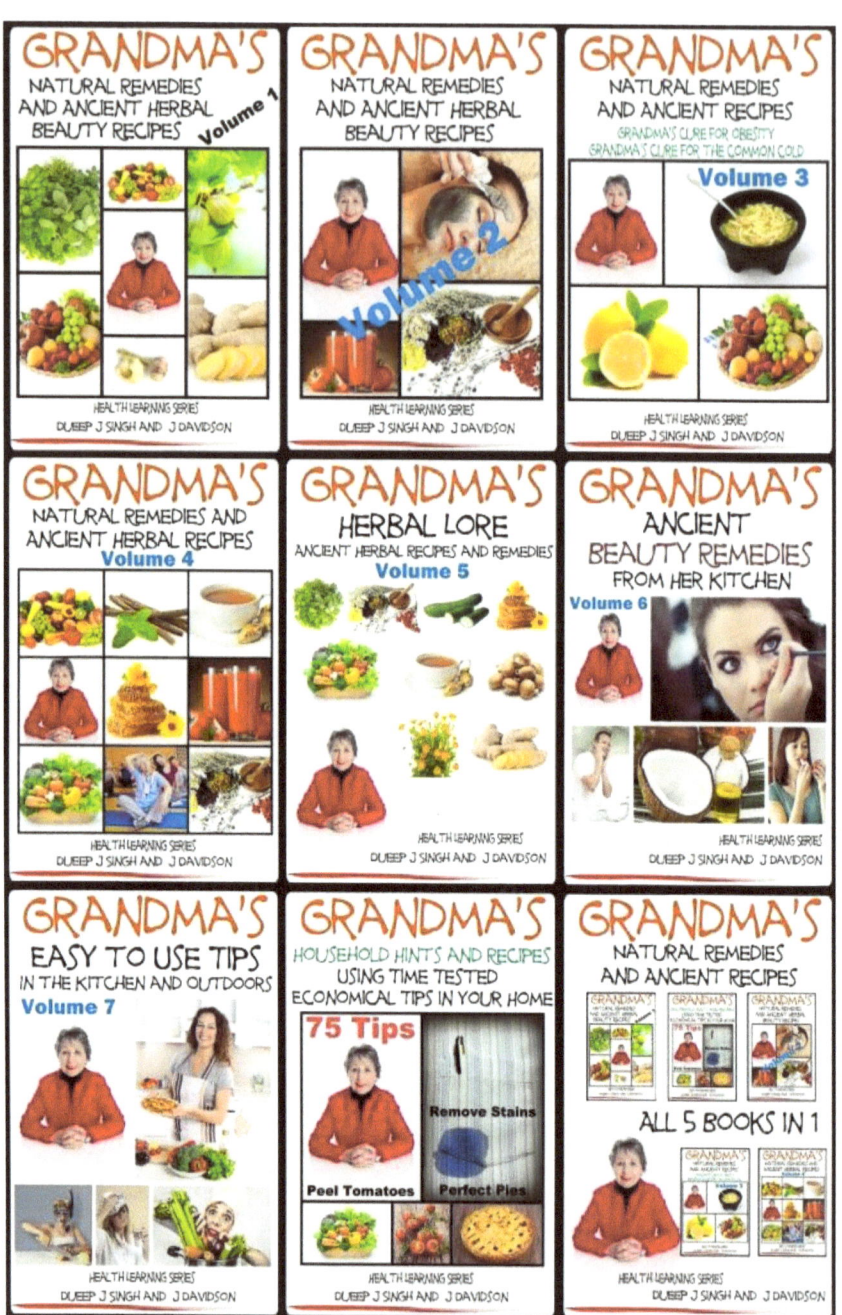

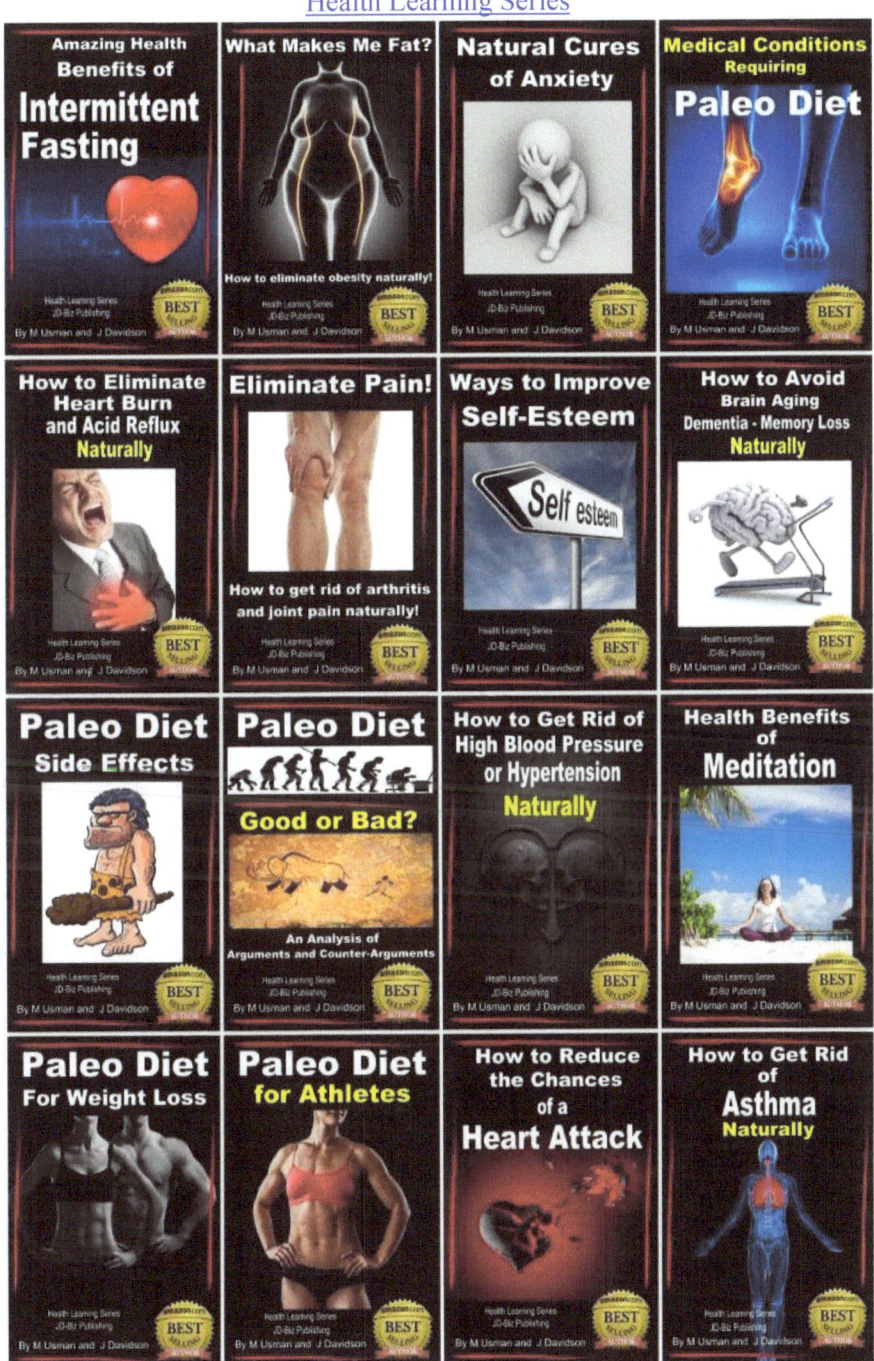

Amazing Animal Book Series

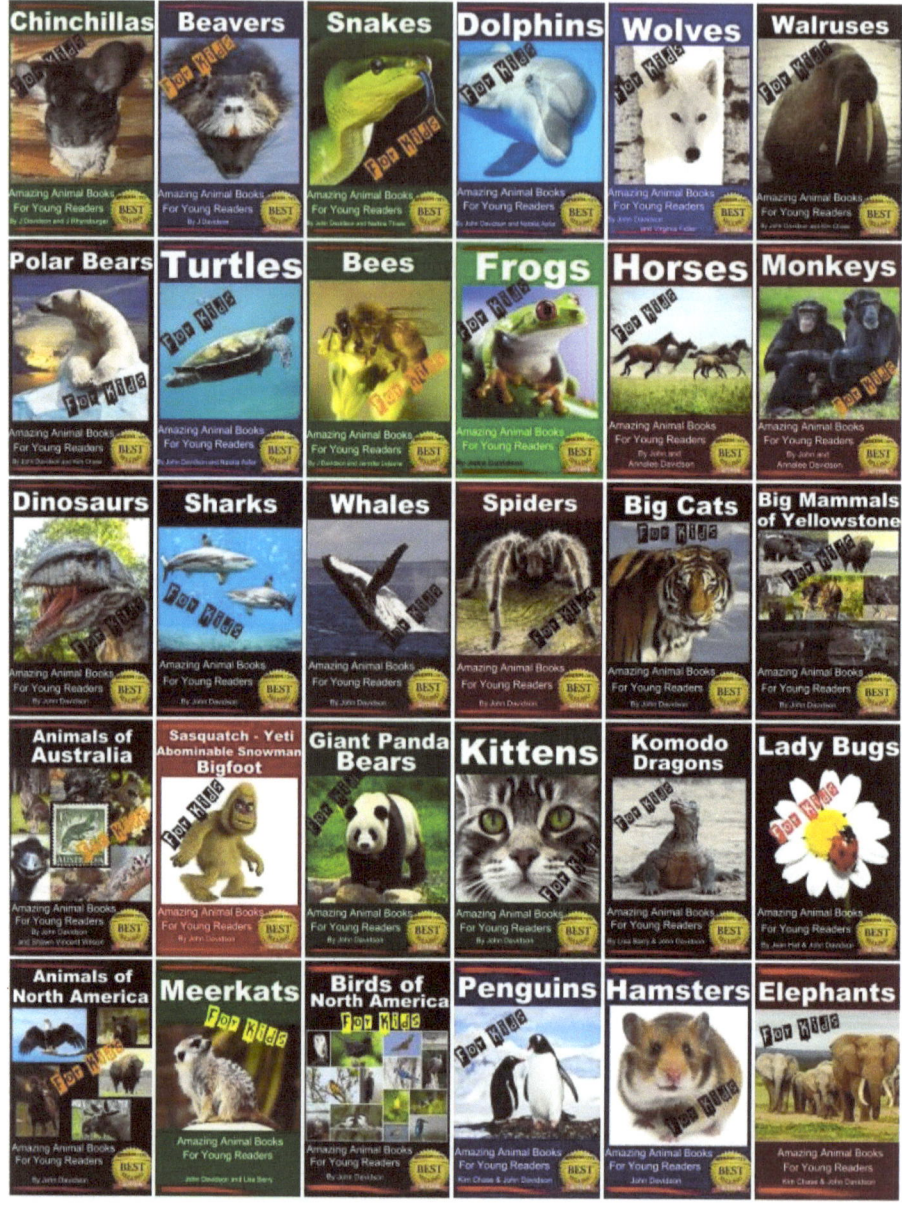

Learn To Draw Series

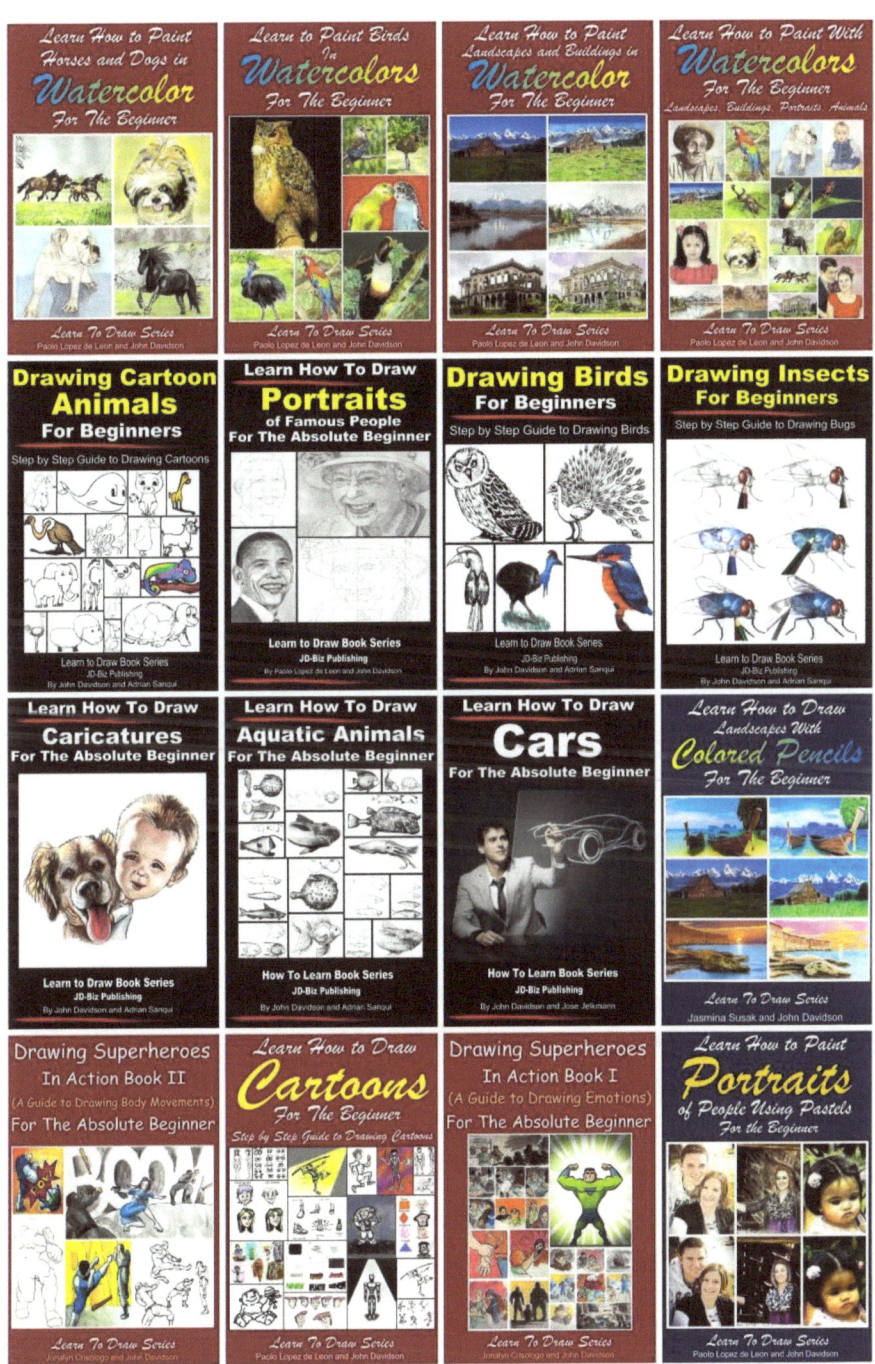

How to Build and Plan Books

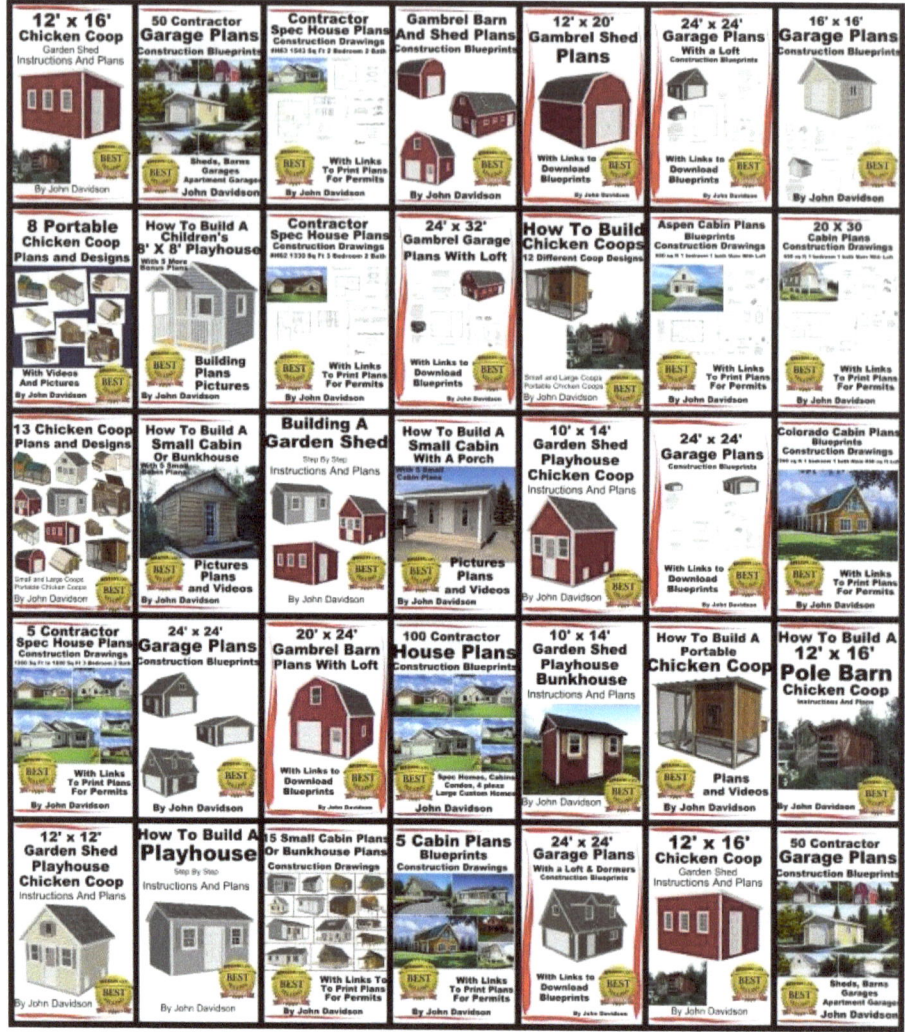

Entrepreneur Book Series

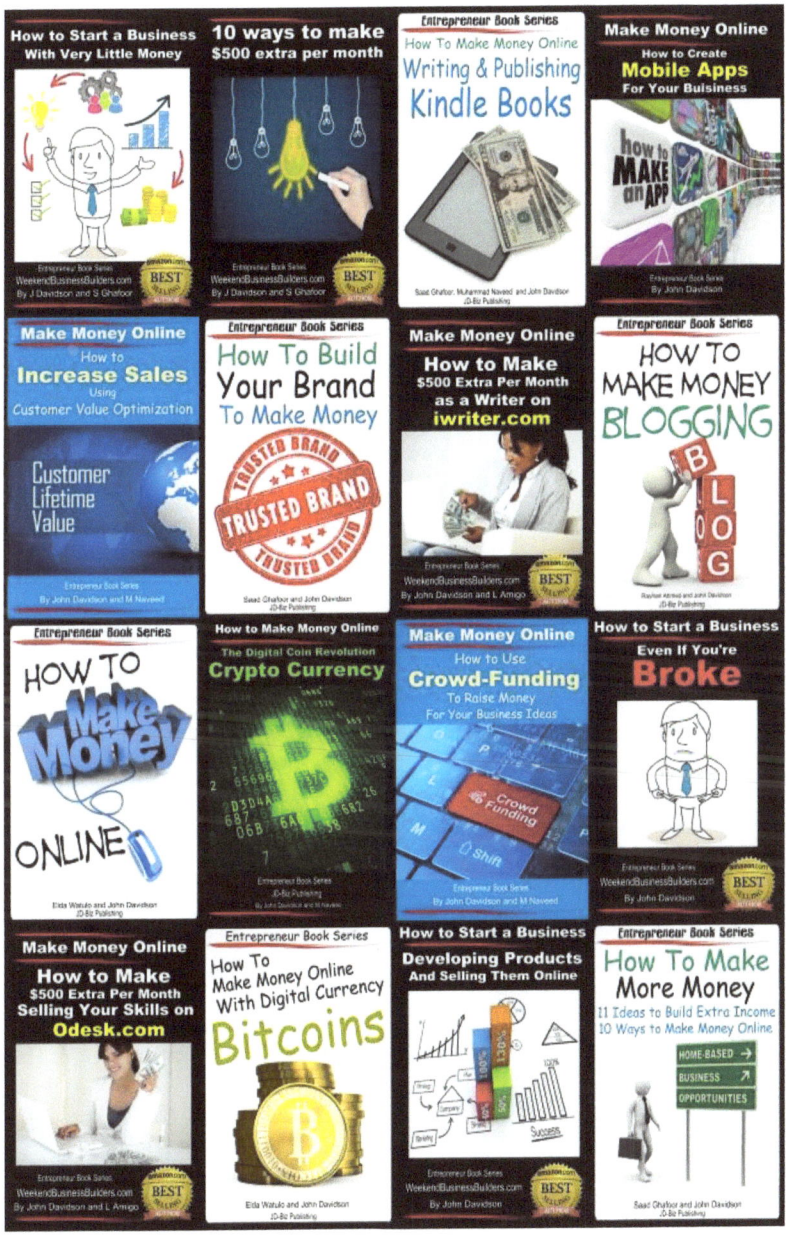

Our books are available at

1. Amazon.com

2. Barnes and Noble

3. Itunes

4. Kobo

5. Smashwords

6. Google Play Books

Download Free Books!

http://MendonCottageBooks.com

Publisher

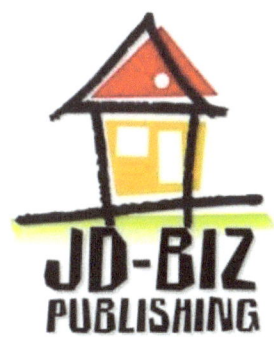

JD-Biz Corp

P O Box 374

Mendon, Utah 84325

http://www.jd-biz.com/

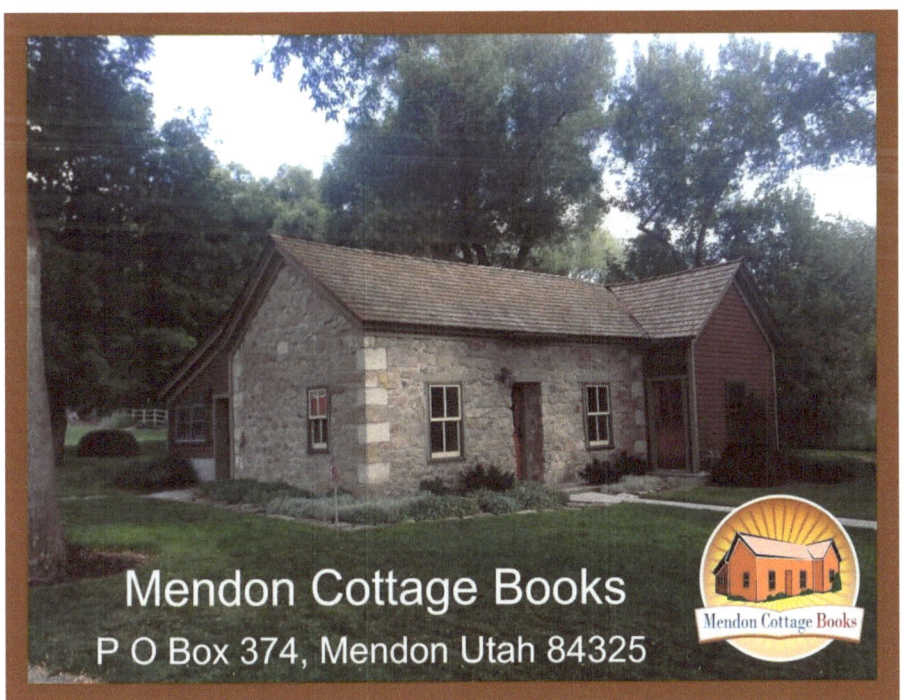

Mendon Cottage Books

P O Box 374, Mendon Utah 84325

www.ingramcontent.com/pod-product-compliance
Lightning Source LLC
Chambersburg PA
CBHW050838290526

45792CB00001B/447